Dr. Lee's Ultimate Guide to a
Rockstar Sexlife
by
Nikeema T. Lee

Copyright © 2015 by Nikeema Lee Publishing
Dr. Lee's Ultimate Guide to a Rockstar Sexlife
Written by Author Nikeema T. Lee
Edited by Upscale Desires Design

ISBN: 978-0990310938 Softcover

All rights reserved. No part of this book may be reproduced or transmitted in any form or by any means, electronic or mechanical, including photocopying, recording, or by any information storage and retrieval system, without permission in writing from the copyright owner.

This book was printed in the United States of America.

ACKNOWLEDGEMENTS

Thank you to all the amazing people who didn't believe that I could win. Thank you to all the men I slept with and all the woman who told me their stories. It is because of you this book was written and its though you that lives will be changed.

To Ainsley Burrows and Laurelle Noel, without your leadership this book would not have been written. Your passion for The Sweet Spot is so incredible. I am GRATEFUL! Thank you for allowing me to dream with you.

To Sabrina Gilbert...boy oh boy... You are such a star. Your smile is my secret wish and I see beauty in it. Thank you for giving me the title of this book and speaking it to life.

Finally IzReal The Poet, thank you for falling in lust with my oral skills. Your bold discovery of one of my many talents lead to me finding my performace family.

                                          Nikeema T. Lee

ROCKSTAR SEXLIFE

FORWARD — 6
INTRODUCTION — 13
CHAPTER 1 — 24
Master who you are
CHAPTER 2 — 32
trust in yourself
CHAPTER 3 — 42
Accept yourself and others
CHAPTER 4 — 49
Are you settling for less
CHAPTER 5 — 60
The language of Sex
CHAPTER 6 — 76
Elevation of Skills
CHAPTER 7 — 84
Demand satisfaction
CHAPTER 8 — 90
Deep Throat
CHAPTER 9 — 98
Beyond Sucking
CHAPTER 10 — 108
Self – Pleasure
CHAPTER 11 — 115
The Best Way to Masturbate for Men
CHAPTER 12 — 132
How to Tantra
CHAPTER 13 — 139
Positions

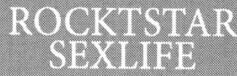

FORWARD

"Sex is a physical expression of your mental, spiritual and emotional condition"

Nikeema T. Lee - American Author

I've dealt with insecurities in my life for a very all time. It was a consistent song in my head. Over and over again, the words of *"you're not enough"* rang in my thoughts. They played since I was eleven years old. That was a time in my life that changed the entire course of my existence. My mother walked out of my life when I was a young girl, leaving a very large whole in my heart that needed to be filled. For years, filling that void was top priority, and by any means necessary. Sex, Drugs and Rock & Roll *wink, were my fillers of choice. I tirelessly poured this deadly mixture into my system. Wanting and craving for my desires to be filled.

This lifestyle landed me in many nights of unfulfilled sexual encounters. I faced countless emotionless stares from people who didn't love me nor wanted to share life's spoils with me. I was just an empty vessel that could be pounded, used, then tossed aside for something fresher and newer.

It was this internal despair that sparked my need to fix my sexual world. Many nights I would find myself lying down with some of the most random men and women. Hoping and praying that this new person would be the one to repair the old wounds of my spirit. Each time given more and more of me away, I became empty and cold. This cycle continued for years and surely I found myself alone and lonely from the inside out.

Knowing that this vicious cycle needed to end, I decide to seek answers. I started reading the latest self-help books and spent thousands of dollars on a coach. I turned within and found my answers. I learned the art of self-reflection and meditation. I believe in the philosophy that sex is just a physical manifestation of what's going on inside. If you fix the inside, the outside will be fixed. The person that is healed and happy on the inside will lead a healed and happy life outside.

With meditation, my sexual world changed. I know what you're thinking, "what does meditation have to do with my sex life? I just want to know how to perform better fellatio or how to squirt." Yes we will discuss those things but its my wish not to put a Band-Aid of your issues. The goal of this book is to lead you to a holistic approach to sexual satisfaction. Who you are inside is a direct reflection of who you will be outside. Your sexlife will remain the same if you remain the same.

Though meditation you can discover truths about yourself. You will uncover the source of your sexual desires. Meditation allows for you to confront the fears associated with a weak sexlife. It answers the questions of lack and helps you to forge into a better, prosperous way of living.

For me through meditation, each day lends to different thoughts. Songs, which sing of love and praises, are now playing in my head because of this practice. Knowing that I deserve the best that life has to offer, pushes me to see past the any situation and into a clear understanding. I am capable of creating a reality beyond my wildest dreams. It's my faith in GOD that keeps me anchored as life looks to toss me about.

THE ART OF MEDITATION

Meditation is not a technique but a way of life. Meditation means 'a cessation of the thought process'. It describes a state of consciousness, when the mind is free of scattered thoughts and various patterns. The observer (one who is doing meditation) realizes that all the activity of the mind is reduced to one.

BREATHING AND MEDIATION EXERCISE
- Seek out a quite place
- Make sure you have a comfortable, straight back chair, or sit with crossed legged on the floor
- Sit quietly for at least 20 minutes
- Take a few minutes to clear your mind
- Take regular breaths
- Clear your mind and concentrate on your breathing
- Relax with every breath

When meditation is first tried, you can easily become distracted and lose sight as to why you're even doing this. A practice like mediation used to center your thoughts and quiet any outside influence is essential to a Rockstar Sexlife. In a state of awareness is where this orgasmic connection can take place. The place where you will find total sexual satisfaction. This intimate meditation should be done everyday to allow for a connection to you and your desires. This peaceful relationship between you and your inner self will allow for you to be at one with your intentions. By designing this level of intimacy in your life daily you will propel yourself closer to a Rockstar Sexlife. 10-20 minutes a day to clear your mind and get grounded to your desires is all you need. For more ways on the benefits and ways to meditate go to www.learning.nikeemalee.com/meditation.

CHAPTER SUMMARY

- Having sexual insecurities in life is OK. Use this book to deal with them.
- Be mindful of what you fill the voids in your life with. For years, filling my void with sex, durg and rock & roll was top priority, and by any means necessary.
- It your internal sexual despair that sparked your need to fix your sexual world.
- Learn the art of self-reflection and meditation.
- With meditation your sexual world will change.
- Though meditation you can discover truths about yourself.
- Daily meditation lends to different thoughts.
- Meditation is not a technique but a way of life.
- A practice like mediation used to center your thoughts and quiet any outside influence is essential to a Rockstar Sexlife.
- By designing this level of intimacy in your life

CHAPTER SUMMARY

daily you will propel yourself closer to a Rockstar Sexlife.
- For more ways on the benefits of meditation go to www.learning.nikeemalee.com/meditation.

INTRODUCTION

> *"Sex pleasure in women is a kind of magic spell it demands complete abandon. If words or movements oppose the magic of caresses, the spell is broken"*
> **Simone de Beauvoir- French Writer**

This book is for you. The one who wasn't born a Sexual Rockstar. The failure and the losers who never found complete satisfaction. Or is it? Ask yourself, are all Rockstars winners? No! Are all of them satisfied? No! Do they never fail? Yes! Rockstars don't always win, many live unfulfilled and most have failed at something. So what makes them different from you? ATTITUDE! It's their attitude about themselves that sets them apart from you. Although Rockstars appear to have this wonderful life, they too have gone through some hardships and heartaches. But though it all they never stop believing the fact they are Rockstars. They've failed. We all have been unsuccessful sexually but the sexual Rockstar never stops trying. They were disappointed and let down but yet still found fullness in their sexlife. They have lost in love perhaps more times then you reading this book yet they found their paths to life's sexual riches.

And so can you...

No longer do you have to settle for less. No longer do you have to push your needs aside for the benefit of someone else. This book will aid you in discovering how to get the most and **BEST** out of your future sexual experiences. You see I said, future experiences, because you can't change the past. You can only live in the present and look forward to the future. This book will allow you to understand how your past sexlife is just that… a thing of your past.

With this book you will;

- Become a Sexual Winner
- Get total satisfaction in your sexlife
- Discover what's been missing in your sexlife
- Find your true orgasmic high
- Find sexual fulfillment every time
- Create mind blowing sexual experiences for years to come!

Are you sick and tired of bad sex? Yes! Disappointing partners? Yes! Unexpected surprises in the bedroom? Yes! Are you tired of waiting for Mr. /Ms. Right to come along so you can share your bed with them? Yes!

GET M.A.D.E.
Master who you are
Accept yourself and others
Demand the best from yourself and others
and
Elevate your skills

Some people **ARE** born Rockstars and others are **MADE**. Don't get caught up on what you weren't born with. Many weren't born the fastest but have a bear chasing you and you will discover speed you didn't even know you had. What's your motavation? Are you being chased by the sexual disappointmnt bear? So what you can't tell if a guy is going to be kind to you once you have sex. Sure you can't tell if a woman will be a porn star in the bed or a lazy Susan before you bought those $300 concert tickets. Not everyone can sense the making of a stalker after you have put the hammer down on someone who can't handle your loving. Use this book to learn the tips, tools and techniques to take your boring, and sometimes scary, sexlife to a soaring sexlife.

- Do you desire to have a sexlife that leaves you smiling and enriched? Read on.
- Do you want to learn how to make your partner moan with ecstasy? Read on
- Do you wish to live a life that sex is the best thing going in your life? Stop reading!

This book is for those seeking to identify why their good pussy or good dick is never kept. How they can have such magic between their thighs yet still be lonely. This book if for the guy that gives his heart to the wrong sister and the woman that trusts the wrong brother. This book is about finding out how you can make lasting connections with any sexual partner that will leave you both enchanted and magically delicious.

SAY GOODBYE TO

- Sexual regrets.
- Bad sexual judgements.
- Lonely nights and,
- "I should've had a V8 moments."

This book is not for people looking to supplement their happiness through sex only. This book will not show you how taking a man's penis deep into your mouth will guarantee that your bills will be paid. This book will not teach you how to make a woman your willing side chick because your tongue game has improved. NO! Stop reading and put this book down. Sex is more than just a means to a financial end. It is more than just a way to emotionally manipulate the weak. It is this low level thinking that leads you to countless nights of sexual regret. This book is not for the people who know that they have been blessed with the tool of the "good dick or good pussy". You don't need this book. You need to bottle what you have and put it on the market so that others can experience the wonder that is you. Haha… F.Y.I. the jokes are scattered throughout this book and they don't get any better than this.

So now that you understand who this book is for and you have decided that this book holds the keys to unlocking mysteries for you, **TAKE ACTION**. So what you have made a connection to the words I have written on the pages. So what it makes you think about your past and the mistakes you have made.
I DONT CARE! Its means nothing if you don't take any action. If you don't apply the tips, tools and techniques offered in this book, your sexlife will continue to be the same. You will

continue to get the same sexual results. Every dollar you spent will be wasted. Don't think you wasted your money on me, oh no. You have wasted your money on yourself. You will also be wasting your time if you don't apply this book to your sexlife. Using this book will take your unfulfilled sexlife and turn you into a sexual Rockstar but it won't if you don't use it.

MAKE THE PROMISE

A promise is a statement telling someone that you will definitely do something or that something will definitely happen in the future. If you promise to apply the tips, tools and techniques outlined in this book, I promise you a Rockstar sexlife. It's that simple. No big commitment. Just do the work. There is a saying that, "everyone wants to live like Diddy but no one wants to work like Puff." Faith without works is dead. These are not my words but the words of the Holy Book. You cannot continue to expect a change in your life and not put in the necessary work to make that change happen, that my friends is called insanity. **STOP** living a crazy life and begin to live the **Rockstar Life**. Start now and make the promise. A promise is also an indication of future success or improvement. This book is an investment in to your future. Bet on yourself. Believe in yourself. Trust in yourself. Get to know yourself.

What do you have to lose? The price of this book, that is all. Ask yourself, "What do I have to gain?" A lifetime of amazing sex and a spirit that is living to its fullest is what awaits you at the end of this book. Don't cheat yourself by not taking action; instead treat yourself to the sweetness of life.

James 2:14-17 New King James Version (NKJV)
Faith Without Works Is Dead

14 What does it profit, my brethren, if someone says he has faith but does not have works? Can faith save him? 15 If a brother or sister is naked and destitute of daily food, 16 and one of you says to them, "Depart in peace, be warmed and filled," but you do not give them the things which are needed for the body, what does it profit? 17 Thus also faith by itself, if it does not have works, is dead.

CHAPTER SUMMARY

- This book is for you, the one who wasn't born a sexual Rockstar, the failure and the losers who never found complete satisfaction.
- Your attitude will determine your altitude to rock stardom
- Reading this book will lead to life's sexual riches
- Forget your sexual past
- With this book you will;
    - Become a Sexual Winner
    - Get total satisfaction in your sexlife
    - Discover what's been missing in your sexlife
    - Find your true orgasmic high
    - Find sexual fulfillment every time
    - Create mind blowing sexual experiences for years to come!
- **GET M.A.D.E.**
    - *Master* who you are
    - *Accept* people for who they are

CHAPTER SUMMARY

- ***Demand*** the best from yourself and others and
- ***Elevate*** your skills
- This book is about finding out how you can make lasting connections with any sexual partner that will leave you both enchanted and magically delicious.
- This book is not for people looking to supplement their happiness through sex only
- Take Action
- Make the Promise

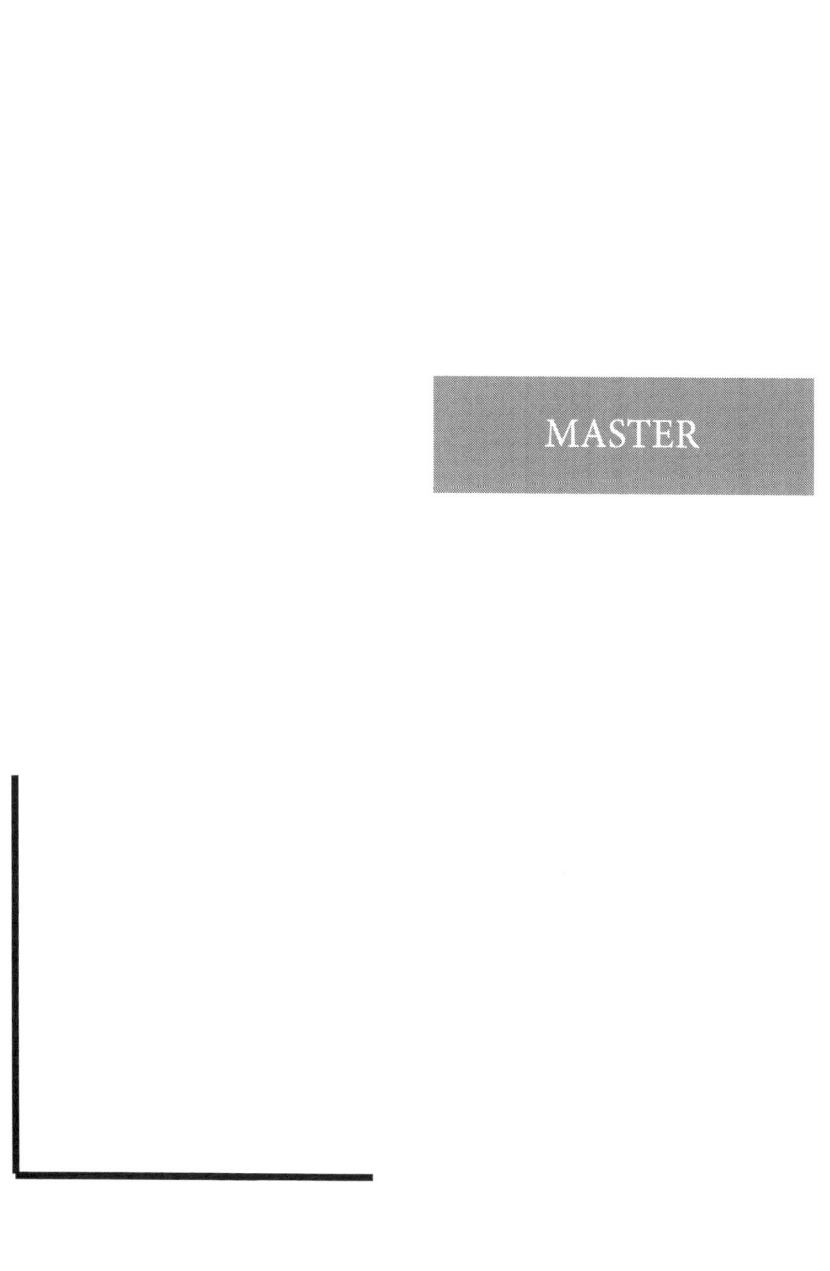

CHAPTER 1

"Love is an ice cream sundae with all the marvelous coverings. Sex is the cherry on top"

Jimmy Dean - American Business Man

MASTER WHO YOU ARE

To Master is to learn (something) completely : to get the knowledge and skill that allows you to do, use, or understand (something) very well. The first step in the M.A.D.E. process to a Rockstar Sexlife is the mastery of yourself. You can't have success with this book if you don't first learn who you are completely.

When it comes to having a Rockstar sex life the most basic thing I can share with you is so simple, but I won't tell you. I mean do you really want know the simple way of creating a great sexlife. Wouldn't you rather hear about how to surfboard on the penis or how to deep throat that thing. I know that those things are what *"you think"* makes sex better. Well I'm here to tell you to get rid of that nonsense. What you do physically is a result of what you think mentally. And what you think of yourself is the most important.

With as many times I've quit or a relationship has ended and yes I've had many relationships end, with each new one, there is still one thing that remains true…sex is important. No matter how old you get, you will continue to have a desire to connect with others, sexually. Love and sex are different. Love is the sundae, sex is the cherry. Great sex begins and ends with love. When you have self love you will always have a Rockstar sexlife.

> *Rule #1*
> *Self-Love is the Best Love*

Self-love has traditionally been seen as a moral flaw, akin to vanity and selfishness. In 1956, however, psychologist and social philosopher Erich Fromm proposed that loving oneself is different from being arrogant, conceited or egocentric, meaning instead caring about oneself, and taking responsibility for oneself is healthy and necessary. Eric Fromm proposed a re-evaluation of self love in a positive sense, arguing that in order to be able to truly love another person, a person needs first to love oneself, in the way of respecting oneself, and knowing oneself (e.g. being realistic and honest about one's strengths and weaknesses)

SELF AWARENESS

Caring about *you* is the first step you can take to developing, maintaining and enhancing your self-esteem, self-worth and self-love. That's right I said self-esteem, self-worth and self-love. How you feel about yourself is a direct reflection on how you will behave sexually. If you feel over weight and don't like the way your skin feels you will be more reluctant to be naked in front of your partner or allow them to freely explore your body.

> *Rule # 2*
> *Great sex starts with you.*

Developing a good relationship with you is essential to an amazing sex life. Many simple steps can be taking to improve your self-image, self-worth and self-love. The one that is by far the best place to start is what you think about yourself. You self-awareness will determine your Rockstar status.

PSYCHOLOGICAL EXERCISE

A major step towards having a Rockstar sexlife and finding a partner to with whom you can truly relate to as an intellectual, sexual and emotional being; is to have confidence in your own mental outlook, physical attractiveness, and emotional status. Before you can develop your self-awareness you must first identify and eliminate the negative pattern of behavior formed by past experiences and replace them with positive and self-enhancing thoughts and attitudes.

To form a loving and giving relationship with another person you must first learn to be at peace with yourself. You must learn to trust yourself. The stress of the day-to-day grind can take a toll on anybody. From the job, to the kids, the twist and turns of life, everything can seem overwhelming. You have to cut yourself off completely from the turmoil of the outside world until you are able to restore yourself both physically and emotionally back to a state of peace and harmony.

The way I suggest you find that is through the psychological exercises of positive thinking. Positive thinking powers the brain cells so that you become more open and alert and allows for you to block out the negativity surrounding your inner being. By developing your positive thinking skills you allow for yourself to be opened from the inside out, given you mental clarity and deeper insight to the inner you.

Positive thinking is a step that can be taking to improve your personal identity. The first step towards finding a loving and fulfilling sexlife is to have a positive attitude towards yourself. How can you expect someone else to love you if you don't love yourself? By following a psychological exercise program each day you can eliminate negative thoughts and accentuate positive ones.

> *Rule # 3*
> *No one will love you unless*
> *you love yourself*

POSITIVITY AFFIRMATION EXERCISE

On one side list some of the things that you feel are negative about yourself. On the other side write positive affirmations that counter that attitude. For examples of Positive affirmation head over to www.learning.nikeemalee.com. There you will find a list of positive vs. negative affirmation that you can use in your daily life.

Negative Thoughts	Positive Affirmations

CHAPTER SUMMARY

- To Master is to learn (something) completely. The first step to a Rockstar Sexlife is the mastery of yourself. You can't have success with this book if you don't first learn who you are completely.
- What you do physically is a result of what you think mentally. And what you think of yourself is the most important.
- Love and sex are different. Love is the sundae, sex is the cherry.
- Rule # 1 Self-Love is the Best Love
- Self love in a positive sense, arguing that in order to be able to truly love another person, a person needs first to love oneself, in the way of respecting oneself, and knowing oneself
- Caring about *you* is the first step you can take to developing, maintaining and enhancing your self-esteem, self-worth and self-love.
- Developing a good relationship with you is essential to an amazing sex life.
- A major step towards having a Rockstar sexlife is finding a partner to with whom you can truly relate as an intellectual, sexual and emotional

CHAPTER SUMMARY

being, is to have confidence in your own mental outlook, physical attractiveness, and emotional status.
- Rule # 2 Great sex starts with you.
- To form a loving and giving relationship with another person you must first learn to be at peace with yourself
- Rule # 3 No one will love you unless you love yourself
- For examples of Positive affirmation head over to www.learning.nikeemalee.com.

CHAPTER 2

"Having sex is all trust. You can't take it back once you do it, and it leaves you completely emotionally vulnerable."

— *Rebecca Donovan, Barely Breathing*

TRUST IN YOURSELF

Soon after I moved to Charlotte, NC to begin my career in radio, I began to doubt whether or not I could do the job. I often wondered if this was the right choice to make. I didn't have a place in the city so I commuted 96 miles one way from Greenville, SC. I traveled back and forth 4 days a week in a car I leased from a friend. I had taken a chance on making this career move and was willing to do what it took to make it work. It just had to work. Boy was it hard to show up and deal with the unexpected work environment while working for a 20% commission of nothing for weeks on end. I noticed that I began to worry and stress about every little thing. From how I was going to put gas in the car to whether my children remember what I looked like. My thoughts began to wonder to the dark side of questioning my abilities, the same abilities that had landed me the job in the first place.

I didn't trust myself. I questioned myself and my decision. Let me explain something, losing control and trusting yourself are difficult things to do. Trust and acceptance - which go hand in hand, are the most powerful tools you have, it is the most potent energy available to you. When you have confidence or, trust, within you, it produces a positive energy that quiets doubt, worry, fear and negative expectations. It has a profound effect on you and others.

When you doubt your power, you give power to your doubt."
– Honore de Balzac

Rule # 4
***Positive energy is more powerful
than negative energy.***

HERE ARE THE 5 THINGS YOU CAN DO TO REBUILD CONFIDENCE IN YOURSELF

- Ground Yourself
- Focus on the positive
- Speak positive
- Take a Break
- Surround yourself with positive people

> *Rule # 5*
> *If you don't trust yourself,*
> *you can't trust others.*

But to trust yourself is also the most empowering decision that you can make. Just think what would happen, if you trusted all your choices and accepted all your decisions - you would be successful in just about everything you do. YES! Everything you do.

Trusting yourself is a learned skill. It requires a deep understanding and acceptance of who you are and what you represent. If I were to ask you, "what do you trust most about yourself?" How would you answer?

The reason you don't trust yourself is because it's a learned emotion, but the actions of others should not affect you. Trusting yourself is about allowing those around you to experience the real you. It's about being authentic. Now - in order to have a Rockstar sexlife experience, you must change it and choose to trust yourself and ***others***.

IT'S TO HARD TO TRUST PEOPLE

I remember the first time someone try to make love to me after my divorce. I was mean and bitter and didn't want anything to do with love. This lead me to have tons of unsatisfying sex. Random and empty. I rejected the idea that someone could love me. I didn't trust them enough to open up. I felt everything he said was a lie. This lack of trust blocked me from reaching my orgasmic high during sex for years. It wasn't until I released the block that my sexlife began to soar. I began to only have sex with people I trusted. This intention helped be to be more open and have a better sexual experiences. If you want to learn how to release the blocks that lead to mistrust go to www.learning.nikeemalee.com.

When people tell you that they love you, believe them. Whether it be an intimate relationship, a friendship, or a family relationship, it is important to accept the declaration of love at face value. If you are pushing aside the gifts of their love because you are afraid that they will hurt you, then you prevent yourself from achieveing sexual satisfication. It also might push them away from you, so that if you change your mind it may be too late.

Ok I know what you're thinking, Nikeema you are crazy to trust people so openly. I would say that your right. So I want you to go back and reread what I said. "I began to only have sex with people I trusted. This intention helped be to be more open and have a better sexual experiences." Having sex with only people I trusted. This trust was build over time. I was lead by my intuition. I trusted myself. I followed my gut. I talked to my potential partner. I asked questions. I shared intimate details about myself and they did the same. So when the topic of sex was brought up, there was a mutual feeling of connection. If someone you met 24 hours ago confesses their sexual connection, this should be your response, "I accept the fact that you want to have sex with me, however I don't feel the same about you at this time." This acknowledgment of their affection allows for you to receive their intentions but it doesn't force you lie about your feelings.

TRUST YOUR A ROCKSTAR

NOW PUT IT ALL TOGETHER

- Trust yourself
- Trust others
- Only have sex with those you trust
- Trust your judgment

When you put all these concept together, as they work together magic will begin to happen. They will wheel wonders in your life by opening your mind and heart to ALLOW love in. Remember sex is only the result of the love. Loving yourself and others and now trusting yourself you can have intense orgasms. There is no internal conversation keeping you from focusing. When your mentally distracted by your fears of lack in love and trust, the only thing to suffer is your orgasm.

CHAPTER SUMMARY

- Trust and acceptance - which go hand in hand, are the most powerful tools you have, it is the most potent energy available to you.
- When you have confidence - or, trust, within you, it produces a positive energy that quiets doubt, worry, fear and negative expectations.
- Rule # 4 Positive energy is more powerful than negative energy.
- 5 things you can do to rebuild confidence in yourself
    - Ground Yourself
    - Focus on the positive
    - Speak positive
    - Take a Break
    - Surround yourself with positive people
- Rule # 5 If you don't trust yourself, you can't trust others.
- Trusting yourself is a learned skill. It requires a deep understanding and acceptance of who you are and what you represent.
- When people tell you that they love you, believe them.

CHAPTER SUMMARY

- Whether it be an intimate relationship, a friendship, or a family relationship, it is important to accept the declaration of love at face value.
- When you put all these concept together, as they work together magic will begin to happen.
  - Trust yourself
  - Trust others
  - Only have sex with those you trust
  - Trust your judgment
- When your mentally distracted by your fears of lack in love and trust, the only thing to suffer is your orgasm.

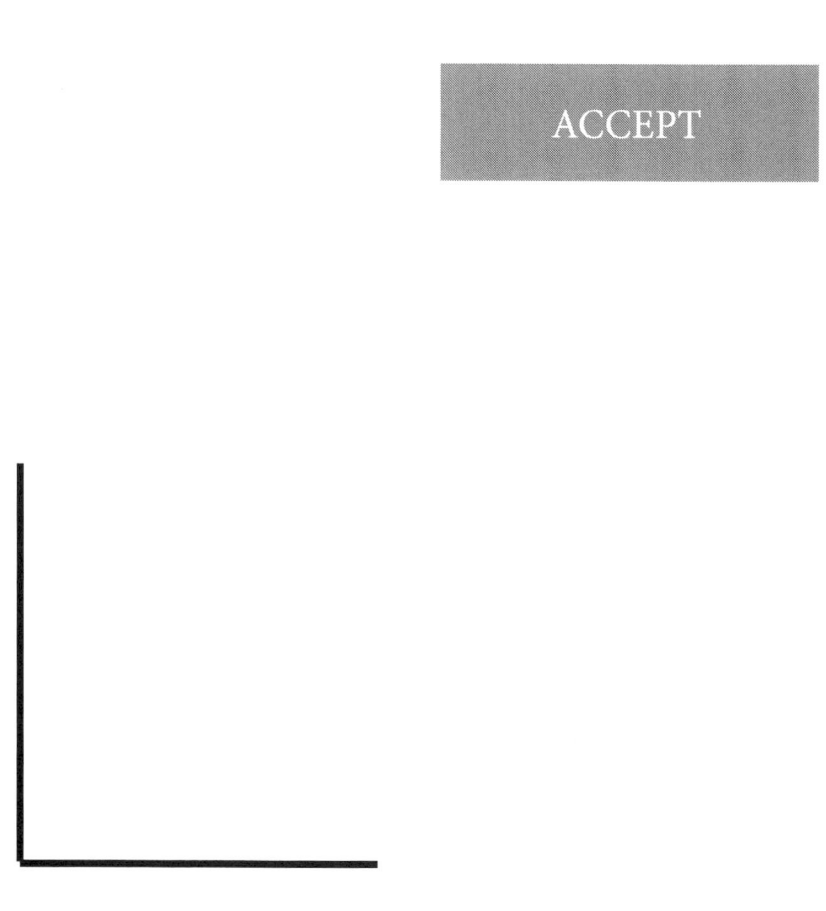

CHAPTER 3

"I don't know the question, but sex is definitely the answer."

Woody Allen, Actor/Movie Director

ACCEPT YOURSELF AND OTHERS

Accept -to take or receive (something offered); receive with approval or favor. Now that we have learned what it takes to master ourselves, let's learn the importance of acceptance This book is written a little differently than you expected I'm sure. Maybe you were looking to just get a few tips you could use in the bedroom. Perhaps you picked up this book looking to become a coochie killer by physically dominating your partner. This book is better.

I would have done you a total disservice if all I offered you was the Band-Aid to a much larger problem. The tips, tools and techniques in this book look way beyond the surface. I aim to penetrate you to your core. I look to reach you way pass your surface and really create a lasting change in your life. I have said this before, "Sex is a physical manifestation of what is going on inside of you;" when you deal only with the outside you get outside results. What are outside results? Think of a rotten banana, its brown, soft and smells. Well even if you take that very same banana and paint it yellow, its still rotten on the inside. Don't continue to live your life as a rotten banana with a fresh coat of paint. You deserve so much more.

> *Rule # 6*
> ***Don't continue to live your life as a rotten banana with a fresh coat of paint.***

That why this book discusses the internal conflicts and obstacles that are preventing you from reaching your highest sexual satisfaction.

BEING M.A.D.E.
In order to have a Rockstar Sexlife you must be M.A.D.E. You must Master, Accept, Demand and Elevate. Here is a small recap. You must Master yourself first before you can master your partner. I will discuss more about your partner's needs in the Elevate part of the book. Accepting is the next goal. Its just as important and equally as difficult. I know I know, you just want to learn about licking and sticking, trust me if you make these internal changes you can become the greatest to ever do it.

This might be the hardest step of all but if you don't accept yourself for who you are; good, bad or ugly, achieving orgasmic bliss will be difficult. Even though its still possible you don't believe that you deserve a sub-standard sexlife, or do you? Do you not deserve to have sexual gratification each and every time you lay with someone? Do you deserve to make lasting and meaningful connections with your sexual partners? If yes, keep reading, If no, start working on why you believe those things by reading my first book; *30 Days to Freedom Becoming*

Authentic: the Ultimate Guide to Falling in Love with the Real you. You can get a copy by going to www.nikeemalee.com. Also practicing the art of meditation will help you explore the reasons, you have difficulty accepting the best of what life has to offer. For more on the benefits of meditation go to www.learning.nikeemalee.com/meditation.

> *Rule # 7*
> *Be willing to Accept Love*

The biggest reason we won't accept ourselves and others is FEAR.

FEARING LOSS.

A common reason for not being able to accept love is prior experience of losing someone you loved, whether it was from death, a break-up, or for some other reason that has scarred you. If you spend all of your life pushing aside love given to you on the off-chance that the person offering it might withdraw it, you will always feel cynical and unsure, which is not a comfortable or happy place to be when it comes to sex. Instead, embrace the love that they are offering and trust yourself, expecting those who offer are being honest. Sometimes its hard to believe someone will be honest with you, I suggest you learn how to be honest with yourself first before you DEMAND it from others. We will talk more about this concept in the next section but first I want to talk about expecting.

The key words is expecting. For some reason many people don't expect to have an orgasm when they have sex. They have become so familiar to unfulfillment that achievement of a heighten state of orgasmic bliss is something they don't even strive for. The road to accepting someone's love in the face of your own fears is a great opportunity to learn the art of allowing. When you can allow YOURSELF to feel love and be loved, you will experience love.

Remember these core prinicples to having a Rockstar sexlife

Love
Trust
Acceptance
Expecting
Allowing
Demanding and
Elevating

CHAPTER SUMMARY

- Accept yourself and others
- The tips, tools and techniques in this book look way beyond the surface. Aimed to penetrate you to your core. Looking to reach you way pass your surface and really create a lasting change in your life
- Rule # 6 Don't continue to live your life as a rotten banana with a fresh coat of paint.
- In order to have a Rockstar Sexlife you must be M.A.D.E. You must Master, Accept, Demand and Elevate.
- This might be the hardest step of all but if you don't accept yourself for who you are; good, bad or ugly, achieving orgasmic bliss will be difficult.
- Rule # 7 Be willing to Accept Love
- **The biggest reason we won't accept ourselves and others is FEAR.**
- A common reason for not being able to accept love is prior experience of losing someone you loved, whether it was from death, a break-up, or for some other reason that has scarred you.

CHAPTER SUMMARY

- Many people don't expect to have an orgasm when they have sex.
- The road to accepting someone's love in the face of your own fears is a great opportunity to learn the art of allowing.
- When you can allow YOURSELF to feel love and be loved, you will experience love.
- Remember these core prinicples to having a Rockstar sexlife
    - Love
    - Trust
    - Acceptance
    - Expecting
    - Allowing
    - Demanding and
    - Elevating

CHAPTER 4

"Sex without love is as hollow and ridiculous as love without sex."

Hunter S. Thompson, American Journalist/Author

ARE YOU SETTLING FOR LESS

When it comes to sex, do you settle or are you just making a bad choice? In this life, every choice matters, and deep in our gut, we know it— this explains why we are sometimes paralyzed over making choices ranging from what to order on a menu to who we should be with in a relationship. When it comes to the choices we make in our sexual relationships; however, so many people choose "settling" for something or someone who is not really what they want. Many say,"Well at least I'm not alone." Yeah you not alone, but you're unhappy, you tell me what is worst.

SETTLING FOR SEX THAT'S LESS THAN WHAT YOU DESIRE IS SIMPLY A BAD CHOICE.

I receive questions each week on my Facebook page, www.facebook.com/nikeemaleecoaching, from women and sometimes men who are desperately trying to figure out a way to have a better sexlife. I ask, "what's wrong with your current sexlife?" Their reply, more often then not is, "my partner just can't please me." This is the crazy thing I have every heard.

> *Rule # 8*
> *You can't be a Rockstar if you settle for less than you desire*

Why would you continue to have sex with someone that doesn't satisfy you? Why make the choice to settle?

You don't have to be an Intimate Relationship Coach or even an expert on love to recognize that fear is what's driving many of these folks to stay in their unhappy situations. Many are willing to do just about anything to avoid an empty house—or an empty bed. Settling for less than what you desire in the bed can only lead to heartbreak and sexual disappointment. You will find yourself asking, "how did this happen to me?" How, you wonder? By settling for something other than what you really, really, truly want and/or desire.

REPEAT AFTER ME
I WANT A ROCKSTAR SEXLIFE

UNDERSTAND THE DIFFERENCE BETWEEN SETTLING AND CHOOSING

First, it's important to understand that the subtle difference between "settling" for bad sex and "choosing" a situation that's best for you. If you feel you settled for bad sex, you could tell yourself you did so because of pressures weighing upon you or fears—in other words, "you had no choice."

However making the choice to continue a situation because its best for you, puts you in control of your own life and the consequences.

> *Rule # 9*
> *Sex is more than physical*

When choosing a situation, take into account more than just your physical pleasure. Here is where your mental, spiritual and emotional equity comes in. You must evaluate if the person stimulates you on a much deeper level. Are you satisfied in the relationship other than your genitals.

Understanding this is one reason we so often avoid making intimate connections with sex partners. We do not fear the sex; we fear what the sex could lead to. Yet, in spite of the fear of the consequences of a bad sex partner, it will always be easier to live with than settling for a situation which makes you unhappy.

Why are you having sex with someone you don't like? Because you're settling for less. If and when you stop settling for less you will receive more. You just have to remember that you are surrounded by abundance, there are more than enough people out there that can give you sexual satisfaction. All you have to do is simply pick! If you don't like what you have, if you don't have what you want, if you want something else just pick something or someone different. Remember that Rockstar's don't settle.

THE WORLD AROUND YOU

Your environment will dictate your direction. If all you can recognize is negative around you or bad sexualmpartner is all you attract, then YOUR around negativity. Remove yourself from it. How? By recognizing the good in your life, by recognizing the joys more than your low.

LOSE THE WEIGHT

Many of us can stand to lose just a few pounds. Don't look at my statement as meaning we all want to be skinny; however, we all want to be fit. Whether it's fit in our bodies or in our minds, having a Rockstar sexlife means having a excited outlook on the possibilities of life.

What happens when you lose more than just the pounds? What happens when the weight of the world begins to lifts off your shoulders? Instead of dropping inches, you're dropping fears.

We think of weight loss as what you burn vs. what you eat. Emotional weight loss is how we love ourselves vs. how we love others. As you continue this journey of Sexual Rock stardom, you will also be losing a different kind of weight.

ROCKSTAR'S ARE M.A.D.E.

Begin to lose things like insecurities, fears and doubts. These compared with pounds, inches and fat will impact your success. Are insecurities, fears and doubts the things holding you back from having a Rockstar Sexlife? Why not lose them to achieve your desires? Why not lose them to achieve greatness? It takes Mastery of self to minimize your ego, live your dreams and face your fears. It will take acceptance to manifest your destiny, courage to demand more for yourself and an elevation of skills to reach new heights.

TAKE TODAY TO

- Master who you are
- Accept yourself and others
- Demand the best from yourself and others and
- Elevate your skills

Rockstar Mantra: I will transform my mind to think differently about myself and the world around me.

We tend to make excuses as to why we are not where we want to be in our sexlives. Why? Its easier to toss blame on others or a condition than to openly acknowledge our own lack of discipline. It take many thing to be successful and have a Rockstar Sexlife; It takes one thing to ruin it all. Excuses!

Excuses are the root of all evil? HAHA nice joke but seriously excuses will completely destroy any hope you could have a for a future. They are monuments to nothingness and bridges to nowhere. When you tend to dish out layers upon layers of excuses as to why we aren't rich or sexually happy, you create a life full of hopelessness and disappointment.

Take back your life today and let go of the fears, and begin to believe again. Find your voice and sing again. The world's greatest orgasm is waiting for you on the other side of that excuse. Will you stop making them in order to succeed? To learn ways you can release insecurities, fears and doubts in your life go to www.learning.nikeemalee.com for my free daily affirmations.

CHAPTER SUMMARY

- When it comes to sex, do you settle or are you just making a bad choice?
- When it comes to the choices we make in our sexual relationships so many people choose "settling" for something or someone who is not really what they want.
- Settling for sex that's less than what you desire is simply a bad choice.
- Rule # 8 You can't be a Rockstar if you settle for less than you desire
- Settling for less than what you desire in the bed can only lead to heartbreak and sexual disappointment.
- Rule # 9 Sex is more than physical
- Making the choice to continue a situation because its best for you, puts you in control of your own life and the consequences.
- We do not fear the sex; we fear what the sex could lead to.
- You just have to remember that you are surrounded by abundance, there are more than enough people out there that can give you sexual satisfaction.

CHAPTER SUMMARY

- Rockstar's don't settle
- Your environment will dictate your direction.
- Whether it's fit in our bodies or in our minds, having a Rockstar sexlife means having a excited outlook on the possibilities of life.
- Emotional weight loss is how we love ourselves vs. how we love others.
- If you want to be a rockstar you must begin to lose things like insecurities, fears and doubts.
- Learn the Rockstar Mantra: I will transform my mind to think differently about myself and the world around me.
- We tend to make excuses as to why we are not where we want to be in our sexlives. Why? Its easier to toss blame on others or a condition than to openly acknowledge our own lack of discipline.
- Excuses are the root of all evil?
- To learn ways you can release insecurities, fears and doubts in your life go to www.learning.nikeemalee.com for my free daily affirmations

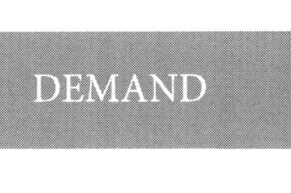

CHAPTER 5

"Anyone who is observant, who discovers the person they have always dreamed of, knows that sexual energy comes into play before sex even takes place. The greatest pleasure isn't sex, but the passion with which it is practiced. When the passion is intense, then sex joins in to complete the dance, but it is never the principal aim."
— *Paulo Coelho,* **Author of The Alchemist**

THE LANGUAGE OF SEX

Despite the prevalence of sexual images in the media, leading to the expectation that having a great sex life is easy, good sexual communication is still one of the most difficult things to achieve in a relationship. Letting one's loved one know what you like in bed requires honesty and patience.

> *Rule # 10*
> ***Demand the best of yourself and others***

The following tips are what you should demand from not only yourself but your potential partner. When you DEMAND the best from yourself and others you pave the way for open communication, deeper connections and heighten sexual experiences. Our sexual desires are real and we must honor them.

One's desires also change over time. Sexual communication is thus an evolving process. Improving how one talks about sex will increase the closeness of the relationship and make it more likely to last! Thus leading to a more powerful orgasmic experience time and time again.

Communication in any relationship is vital. Sexual communications even more so then often the hardest thing to do. We are generally given no tools for this and end up doing things we don't enjoy or are not getting what we want sexually because we don't know how to ask for it. Often we feel embarrassed about expressing our desires for fear of what our partner will think or how they'll respond. We also don't want to hurt their feelings.

This lack of communication leads to dissatisfaction with sexuality, which in turn causes its own problems. It also creates a situation of general unhappiness about not being able to fully express yourself in life. It's important to understand that as fearful as you are of opening up sexually, your partner is probably just as nervous as you.

KNOWING ONE DOESN'T KNOW EVERYTHING

Every woman and man is unique in terms of how they like to be touched. Even if one has a wealth of sexual experience, one may not understand how this particular partner feels. Some enjoy rough play; some gentle. Some like frequent sex; some irregular intercourse. Some women can orgasm with mild manual stimulation; some require the use of sex toys. Not presuming one knows what one's partner likes is the first step to asking them what they want.

ASKING THE RIGHT QUESTIONS

Begin by touching your partner gently and, while you're doing so, asking them what they like. Do you enjoy having your nipples squeezed? Do you like your neck nibbled? Is this enough pressure on your clitoris? Are deep thrusts comfortable for you?

Once they let one know what they appreciate in bed, remember, this doesn't mean that one's range of sexual desires doesn't have to be reviewed throughout a relationship. It does mean that one's partner wants to feel heard. It can be annoying and a turn-off to have to answer questions every time one has sex. Even more frustrating is feeling that the lover wasted her time letting a partner know what she likes only to have him forget!

A USEFUL TECHNIQUE

The following technique makes this communication much easier and allows you to guide a discussion without putting any pressure on your partner. Asking your partner HOW something feels or what he/she likes or doesn't enjoy puts pressure on them.

- Firstly they have to describe something that they may be embarrassed about.
- Secondly many people will not say something negative for fear of offending or upsetting their partner.

The simplest and best way to begin talking about something sexual is to ask questions that require your partner to answer

YES or NO, nothing else.

- You can do this during lovemaking or afterwards.
- In fact, in a neutral time and place may be even safer.

Here's an example of how this works. Let's use the issue of caressing your partner's nipples.

'Do you like the way I touch your nipples?' 'Would you like me to kiss your nipples more?'

'Would you like me to kiss your nipples firmer, more gently, more on the sides etc?' 'Would you like me to kiss your nipples softer?'

This allows you to learn lots about what your partner wants and how to please them in a very gentle way. If you're doing this during sex then the conversation can be a little different. As you touch your partner you ask them for feedback. Let's use the same example as before.

Kiss the nipple in a particular way and ask:

Does this feel good, would you like me to do this harder, softer, faster, or slower?'

Each time you ask a question and do something different wait for them to answer. You can also allow your partner to guide you by using simple words, harder, softer, slower, faster, left, right, up or down. This way you're able to avoid negative criticism about what they're doing.

BEING OPEN MINDED AND NON-JUDGMENTAL

Along with feeling heard, most people want to feel that their desires are normal, or at least acceptable. Some people enjoy being tied up during sex, or like visual stimulation, or appreciate the use of a range of toys. Even if one isn't experienced in this practice, the worst response one can have is disgust, shock or other signs that you are disturbed by their desires. If one loves or cares about the person, one will want them to feel good in the way that makes them happy. While one doesn't have to do anything that makes one feel comfortable, neither should anyone make a loved one feel odd or unclean for enjoying those forms of arousal. Most importantly, make all sexual partners feel good about their bodies and never draw attention to their flaws. Being criticized for things one cannot change is the ultimate turn-off.

Because sex is so important to us, as is the image of being a

Rockstar lover, when we get told negatively what we're doing wrong we tend to withdraw. I'm afraid to say that we all are at fault here, thinking we know everything, particularly about sex. But here's a fact, the only way we know if something feels good and pleasurable is to ask.

It's important to respect your partner's communication and guidance. This will build deep trust and safety between you. This gentle approach opens the door to communicating about other areas of life as well. You'll also find that after doing this a few times it will be easier to talk about sex in a more open and honest way.

MAINTAINING CARE AND TRUST

Here is that word again---TRUST. I cannot emphasis enough how important trust is to having a Rockstar Sexlife. If an individual feels that his partner really cares about them, they more likely to be able to tell her what he likes. You are more likely to be more open, accepting and allowing. Knowing that one's significant other wants to listen, learn and expand the pleasures of one's sex life will increase the openness. A solid level of trust helps one to feel that they won't share this information with others outside the relationship, betray you or deliberately hurt you. Sexual communication is sure to improve and with it, the overall quality of the relationship and orgasm.

INTIMACY

Dr. Henry Brandt, in the Collegiate Challenge magazine, said that there is a syndrome, a pattern, when couples come to him. They say, "At first, sex was exciting. Then I started feeling funny about myself, and then I started feeling funny about my partner. We argued and fought and finally we broke up. Now we are enemies." This syndrome is called the morning-after syndrome. We wake up and find that intimacy is not really there. The sexual relationship does not satisfy us anymore, and what we end up with is not what we really wanted in the first place. All you have is two self-centered people seeking self-satisfaction. The elements of genuine love and intimacy cannot be obtained "instantly," and you find yourself in an unbalanced state, searching for harmony.

Each of us has five significant parts in our lives. We have the physical, the emotional, the mental, the social, and the spiritual. All five of these parts are designed to work together in harmony. In our search for intimacy we want the solution today, or yesterday. One of our problems is that we want "instant" gratification. When the need for intimacy in a relationship is not met, we look for an "instant" solution. Where do we look? Physical, mental, social, emotional or spiritual? It's the physical. It is easier to be physically intimate with someone than to be intimate in any of the other four areas. You can become physically intimate with a person of the opposite sex in an hour, or half-hour -- it just depends upon the urge! But you soon discover that sex may only be a temporary relief for a superficial desire. There is a much deeper need that is still unmet.

What do you do when the thrill wears off and the more you have sex, the less you like it? All across America, men and women are searching for intimacy, going from one relationship to another hoping, "This time will be it. This time I am going to find a relationship that will last."

I believe that what we really want is not better sex. What we really want is true intimacy. The key to a Rockstar Sexlife is find true intimacy in your relationship BEFORE you have a phsycial relationship with them. Now you understand my you must be walked through certain steps. Read on.

WHAT IS INTIMACY?

Today, the word intimacy has taken on sexual connotations. But it is much more than that. It includes all the different dimensions of our lives -- yes, the physical, but also the social, emotional, mental and spiritual aspects as well. Intimacy really means total life sharing. And haven't we all had the desire at one time or another for closeness, for oneness, for sharing our life with someone totally?

Marshall Hodge wrote a book called Your Fear of Love. In it he says, "We long for moments of expressions of love, closeness and tenderness, but frequently, at the critical point, we often draw back. We are afraid of closeness. We are afraid of love." Later in the same book Hodge states, "The closer you come to somebody, the greater potential there is for pain.*"It is the fear of pain that often drives us away from finding true intimacy."*

I would estimate that around 100 percent of the population would say you have been hurt in a relationship before. The question is how do you handle that hurt? We build walls around our hearts to protect us from anyone on the outside getting in to hurt us. But that same wall which keeps people out, keeps us stuck inside. The result? Loneliness sets in and true intimacy and love become impossible.

In human relationships, the meaning and level of intimacy varies within and between relationships. In anthropological research, intimacy is considered the product of a successful seduction, a process of rapport building that enables parties to confidently disclose previously hidden thoughts and feelings. Intimate conversations become the basis for 'confidences' (secret knowledge) that bind people together.

Developing an intimate relationship typically takes a considerable amount of time (months and years, rather than days or weeks) and both anthropologists and zoologists have tracked the subliminal changes in body language as rapport develops between two or more people.

To sustain intimacy for any length of time requires well developed emotional and interpersonal awareness. Get my free guide to sustaining intimacy at www.learning.nikeemalee.com. Intimacy requires an ability to be both separate and together participants in an intimate relationship. From a center of self-knowledge and self-differentiation intimate behavior joins family, close friends as well as those with whom one is in love. It evolves through reciprocal self-disclosure and candor. Poor skills in developing of intimacy can lead to getting too close too quickly; struggling to find the boundary and to sustain connection; being poorly skilled as a friend, rejecting self-disclosure or even rejecting friendships and those who have them. The more time used to develop your intimacy with your partner the greater result you will have when connecting with your partner and creating the Ultimate Rockstar Sexlife.

CHAPTER SUMMARY

- Despite the prevalence of sexual images in the media, leading to the expectation that having a great sex life is easy, good sexual communication is still one of the most difficult things to achieve in a relationship.
- Rule # 10 Demand the best of yourself and others
- When you DEMAND the best from yourself and others you pave the way for open communication, deeper connections and heighten sexual experiences.
- Improving how one talks about sex will increase the closeness of the relationship and make it more likely to last!
- Communication in any relationship is vital. Sexual communications even more so then often the hardest thing to do.
- This lack of communication leads to dissatisfaction with sexuality, which in turn causes its own problems.
- It's important to understand that as fearful as you are of opening up sexually, your partner is probably just as nervous as you.

CHAPTER SUMMARY

- The simplest and best way to begin talking about something sexual is to ask questions that require your partner to answer YES or NO, nothing else.
- Along with feeling heard, most people want to feel that their desires are normal, or at least acceptable.
- If an individual feels that his partner really cares about them, they more likely to be able to tell her what he likes. You are more likely to be more open, accepting and allowing.
- The elements of genuine love and intimacy cannot be obtained "instantly," and you find yourself in an unbalanced state, searching for harmony.
- Today, the word intimacy has taken on sexual connotations. But it is much more than that. It includes all the different dimensions of our lives -- yes, the physical, but also the social, emotional, mental and spiritual aspects as well.
- *It is the fear of pain that often drives us away from finding true intimacy."*
- In human relationships, the meaning and level of intimacy varies within and between relationships.
- To sustain intimacy for any length of time requires

CHAPTER SUMMARY

well developed emotional and interpersonal awareness.
- more time used to develop your intimacy with your partner the greater result you will have when connecting with your partner and creating the Ultimate Rockstar Sexlife.

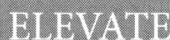

CHAPTER 6

"Clinton lied. A man might forget where he parks or where he lives, but he never forgets oral sex, no matter how bad it is."

Barbara Bush - Former First Lady of the United States of America

ELEVATION OF SKILLS

WOW!! What a ride. You have explored so much about yourself. Mastering, Accepting and Demanding. For my free guide to the Art of Allowing go to www.learning.nikeemalee.com. You are 95% of the way to having a Rockstar Sexlife. Yes sex is 95% mental, spiritual and emotional and only 5% physical. Now that we have address the issues that block you from trusting and accepting, we can get to the deliciousness of sex. The sweaty, raw and intoxicating part of sex. Elevating your skills is the final step to having a Rockstar sexlife. I love this part of the book and will start me my favorite topic.

FELLATIO!

How many dick suckers are reading this? Haha... If hearing that word makes you blush or offended then you shouldn't be having sex at all. This book is meant to help you lose the last bit of obstacles that can be holding you back from opening up completely. Knowing more about your partner is nothing compared to learning more about yourself. Now back to our lesson in oral stimulation.

The Blowjob

There isn't a man alive who wouldn't sell his soul for an amazing blowjob. You may feel that you already have a killer head game, and I have no doubt you do, however you may read on a find a few tips that will help catapult your Mic skills to new heights. If you're a beginner, read the tips and choose two or three suggestions you would like to try. Remember not ever tip, tool and technique is for you and will bring pleasure to your partner, so try them all and PRACTICE, PRACTICE, PRACTICE.

> *Rule # 11*
> *Practice, Practice, Practice*

Also take into account that as we get older and have different sexual partners, our needs will change and evolve so if you have been in a relationship for a significant amount of time trying something new for your partner may open uncharted doors that can lead to great sexual satisfaction. I know that many of you participate in then act and wonder how you can improve on your performance. Well this book is here to show you a few tips that you need to have in order to take your blowjob skills to Rockstar status.

MASTER YOUR PARTNER

Mastering your partner is simply…learning them.

THE ANATOMY

Do you know all the parts of the penis? I bet you don't. Test your knowledge by matching the parts of the penis to their description.

Glans	The area between the anus and the testicles
Frenulum	Where sperm is made and stored for ejaculation
Shaft	The most sensitive part of the penis
Perineum	The Head of the penis
Testicles	The length of the penis

Check the Chapter Summary for the answers. How did you do? Do you know your penis?

Rate of score

0-1: you are penis **NOVICE** and I believe you may even be a virgin. It's completely OK. However this book may make you into a complete expect by the time you are finish

2-4: you are a **PRO** and you know your penis. Keep reading for a great way to use your knowledge

5: You are an **EXPECT** on all things male reproduction and your knowledge of your partner is going to make you a bona fide Rockstar in no time, so keep reading.

So now that you know the anatomy of your partner, get to know then personally. Please note that every man is different and will experience different things with different woman for different reasons. Don't get so wrapped up in a technique that you can't give your partner pleasure because you have the moves of Peter and Tom mastered but you're now with Phil and he desires something totally different. When you take the time to learn what your current partner needs, wants and or desires you are 95% of the way to Rockstar status with your current mate.

Blowjobs aren't just for men's pleasure. Many women say the feeling of control and power combined with the pleasure she can give is a complete turn on. So in order to find pleasure for both you and your partner ask him if receiving a blowjob is something he desires. Some men hold different beliefs on the act and you may have stumbled upon one that has no desire to have is flesh slurped up by your vacuum jaws. So instead of wasting your mouth mileage on someone who would otherwise not receive this oral pleasure, ask them what they want.

By asking your partner you learn two things:
Whether you can or can't meet his demands.

You will have a clear picture of what the mandate on your time will be in order to pleasure your partner. A mature and honest man should be able to communicate his needs and desires to you. If you're not sure what kind of man you have, please take my free personality quiz at www.learning.nikeemalee.com.

ACCEPT THE CHALLENGE
Now that you have asked and he has answered, you can now ACCEPT or DECLINE the job. Get it... Blowjob! It's not just a casual thing. Remember that you are putting someone penis into your mouth. Now the penis is not the cleanest thing in the world. Men are dirty and the penis is no exception. Even

the cleanest man can have sweaty, uncircumcised and even down right smelly penis any time of the day. Well maybe not uncircumcised but you get my point, you never know what you going to get. So knowing and accepting your level of commitment is essential. When you agree to accept your partner's needs you are accepting all of them. Making a full effort to provide your partner with a full array of the things they need is important to having a healthy relationship. You are either all in or all out.

> *Rule # 12*
> ***Never suck a dick you don't like***

That's why rule number 12 is important. The best head involves a giver who is totally into it, someone who is even aroused by doing it. So if you don't like, trust or believe in your partner, why suck their penis? Are you doing it for some other low level reason? Are you doing it so he will like you? Are you doing it so that you can keep him around? If you answered yes to any of these questions please go to www.learning.nikeemalee.com so that you can learn tools and techniques to loving yourself and destroy the underlying issues that have brought you to this level of thinking.

CHAPTER SUMMARY

- This book is meant to help you lose the last bit of obstacles that can be holding you back from opening up completely.
- PRACTICE, PRACTICE, PRACTICE.
- Mastering your partner is simply…learning them.
- Do you know your penis?
  - Glans -The Head of the penis
  - Frenulum- The most sensitive part of the penis
  - Shaft-The length of the penis
  - Perineum-The area between the anus and the testicles
  - Testicles-Where sperm is made and stored for ejaculation
- Please note that every man is different and will experience different things with different woman for different reasons.
- When you take the time to learn what your current partner needs, wants and or desires you are 95% of the way to Rockstar status with your current mate.
- Blowjobs aren't just for men's pleasure. Women enjoy the power of pleasing their mate.
- By asking your partner you learn two things:
  - Whether you can or can't meet his demands.

CHAPTER SUMMARY

- A mature and honest man should be able to communicate his needs and desires to you.
- Penis sucking not just a casual thing. We are talking about putting human flesh into your mouth. Knowing and accepting your level of commitment is essential.
- When you agree to accept your partner's needs you are accepting all of them. Making a full effort to provide your partner with a full array of the things they need is important to having a healthy relationship. You are either all in or all out.
- If you don't like, trust or believe in your partner, why suck their penis?
- Are you doing it for some other low level reason? Are you doing it so he will like you? Are you doing it so that you can keep him around? If you answered yes to any of these questions please go to www.learning.nikeemalee.com so that you can learn tools and techniques to loving yourself and destroy the underlying issues that have brought you to this level of thinking.

CHAPTER 7

"If sex were shoes, I'd wear you out. But I wouldn't wear you out in public."

— *Jarod Kintz, American Author*

DEMAND SATISFACTION

Now I'm talking to my people who have a worship of the penis and it's justified. You must find it extremely erotic to pleasure your partner in this way. You must enjoy the feeling of penis in your mouth, how it looks in your hands and how it stimulates you tongue. Getting off on the feeling of power you have over your lover as you control his pleasure, should give you a sexual charge and ultimately make you orgasm when you perform it. Whatever your drive, you must absolutely, positively be into giving this man the best blowjob of his life each and every time you perform, otherwise no one will enjoy it. It will be a complete waste of your mouth mileage and his penis time. Use your time wisely.

When it comes to giving head there are guidelines to performing it at the Rockstar level. You can take your skills to one man or many men and quickly determine what will work best for him.

> *Rule # 13*
> *Giving Head saves lives*

GIVE HEAD

Studies have proven that women who perform fellatio at least 2-3 times a week live a longer life. Now experts can determine whether it's the act itself or the heartfelt enjoyment that leads to a longer life. I believe in the latter. I believe that it's the joy that women get from pleasing her man in such a way that it gives her satisfaction. Performing the act of fellatio regularly is not only beneficially for the woman but it also helps to enhance the relationship bring couples together on a deeper intimate level more often.

EXPLORE HIS WHOLE BODY

Starting slow by touching, licking and kissing him will alert his brain that something is about to go down. Don't be afraid to explore is other pleasure zones like his nipples before heading to the targeted area. Being vocal also never hurt. Talking dirty to him is a great way to help focus your mind on the task at hand and gets him aroused quickly. The idea is to let him know you are really into doing this deed for him and to him.

USE YOUR WHOLE BODY

The best blowjob involve more than just your mouth, and focus on much more than just his penis. Use everything he has to please him. Again by using your whole body you show him that you are just as into the giving as he is into the receiving. Use not just your mouth but also your tongue, face, hair, hands, nails and even chest to heighten his experience. Rubbing is penis against your vagina can be the ultimate stimulator but be careful not to get to carried away that you stick it in and forget to actually perform fellatio. Try not to over think your movements and let your body and mind get in sync with the rhythm of his body naturally.

START SLOW

When you first encounter his penis, remember to move slowly. Take your time and get acquainted with it. If it's flaccid, and it shouldn't be if you have employed the skills from above, however if you have skipped those steps go back and use them, they are important to giving a Rockstar blowjob. With your hands, mouth and tongue, explore every inch of his stiffness. Run your tongue along his shaft, remembering to give a little eye contact in the process. This will help to maintain the intimate connection you are looking to build by doing this in the first place.

BE CREATIVE

There is no exact play by play that you must to do, so allow yourself to be swept away in the magic energy of your work. You are the painter and his penis is your canvas. Lick and suck your way to a masterpiece. Run your tongue along his shaft, noting the texture of each vein and bulge. Run your tongue along is testicles, placing them in your mouth and sucking them. Monitor his responses so you know what he likes without him even having to tell you. Try to move seamlessly from his shaft to the head of his penis. Make your movement effortless. Every man is different; the same man might love a gentle touch one night and may want you to bite his penis another…literally "bite my penis." Don't be afraid to try something new. If he likes it, his body will let you know. If he doesn't, just pay attention and move on to something else.

CHAPTER SUMMARY

- You must enjoy the feeling of penis in your mouth, how it looks in your hands and how it stimulates you tongue. Getting off on the feeling of power you have over your lover as you control his pleasure, should give you a sexual charge and ultimately make you orgasm when you perform it.
- Whatever your drive, you must absolutely, positively be into giving this man the best blowjob of his life each and every time you perform, otherwise no one will enjoy it.
- GIVE HEAD Studies have proven that women who perform fellatio at least 2-3 times a week live a longer life.
- Rule # Giving Head saves lives
- Explore His Whole Body. Starting slow by touching, licking and kissing him will alert his brain that something is about to go down.
- Use your Whole Body. The best blowjob involve more than just your mouth, and focus on much more than just his penis.

CHAPTER SUMMARY

- Start Slow. When you first encounter his penis, remember to move slowly. Take your time and get acquainted with it.
- Be Creative. There is no exact play by play that you must to do, so allow yourself to be swept away in the magic energy of your work. You are the painter and his penis is your canvas.

CHAPTER 8

"The main reason Santa is so jolly is because he knows where all the bad girls live."

— George Carlin, American Comedian

DEEP THROAT

We will get back to more tips for penis pleasure. The topic of deep throating is so intense it had to get it's own chapter. Be slick at this point and add your personal lubrication to his penis. Don't waste your time finding silicone based lubes or something flavored. You can produce all that you need in order to grasp the ultimate Rockstar experience. The process of deep throating his penis is a complete turn on for him. Seeing you take a large part if not all of his penis into your mouth will send electric charges through his body and make you the ruler of his penis.

THE THROAT

If you want to relax your throat, guess what, drinking alcohol will not help. Alcohol actually tightens the throat muscles. This is especially true for spirits, so steer clear if you want to have an enjoyable experience. Many have long believe that getting drunk will help you have a better time while having sex, when in fact it takes away from the wonderful feeling. Besides, if you're a bit on the tipsy side you may not be aware of whether or not if he is actually enjoying your performance!

Another great technique is to breath. As penis goes further down your throat your ability to exchange carbon dioxide for oxygen is limited. If you want to breathe do it through your nose.

Finally, get that throat wide open. The best technique to do this is to exhale. Remember to exhale *before* you take his penis in your mouth. This will increase your oral capacity by about 33%. Try it. Take a deep breath in. Notice that the tongue draws itself up and in. Now exhale, see how the mouth opens up and relaxes.

Now let's tackle the ugly elephant in the room, the dreaded gag reflex. When deep throating the penis you will inevitable encounter the dreaded gag reflex. The pharyngeal reflex or gag reflex (also known as a laryngeal spasm) is a reflex contraction of the back of the throat. It's evoked by touching the roof of the mouth, the back of the tongue, the area around the tonsils and the back of the throat. The gag reflex prevents something from entering the throat except as part of normal swallowing and helps prevent choking.

Because our bodies are built for survival the brain will sense the trigger of your gag reflex as a call for help and in doing so will produce saliva in order to help free the throat from the obstruction. This nature pool of lube can be used to help you take his penis further down your throat.

As a deep throat expert I have listed the

TOP 10 WAYS YOU CAN REDUCE YOUR GAG REFLEX FOR A BETTER FELLATIO EXPERIENCE:

1. Numb your soft palate. When an object touches the soft palate (far back in the roof of your mouth), it can trigger the gag reflex, so you can use a numbing throat spray to desensitize the soft palate, or a gel that's normally used to relieve tooth pain. The effects should last for about an hour, and your soft palate will be less reactive.

2. Disengage your gag reflex. By gradually getting your soft palate accustomed to being touched, you can minimize the gag reflex, or perhaps even get rid of it completely. This is the first step that sword swallower must take and it does require effort and patience over time.

3. Relax. The gag reflex is triggered by a combination of psychology and physiology. For some people, the psychological aspect will play a larger role. Maybe you've had a traumatizing experience at a doctor or dentist's office in the past, or in general, you have a fear of losing control. Some steps such as controlled breathing, will help. You may also want to practice some form of meditation. In more extreme situations, some people find hypnosis works.

4. Lift both of your legs if you're sitting or lying down on your back. Tightening your abdominal muscles might help stop gagging.

5. Make a fist. Close your left thumb in your left hand and make a fist. Squeeze tight.

6. Put a little table salt on your tongue. Moisten the tip of your finger, dip it into some salt, and dab the tip of your tongue with that. Another way to do this is to put a teaspoon of salt in a glass of water, and rinse your mouth with that. Don't forget to spit!

7. **Hum.** You might find that it's difficult to gag and hum at the same time.

8. Listen to music. Distracting your mind can help keep it from giving too much focus to that which gags you.

9. Beware the gag reflex in the morning. Some people report that they're more likely to gag earlier in the day. Try to schedule the gag-inducing activity for the late afternoon or evening instead.

10. Breathe through your nose. Taking a nasal decongestant beforehand can help clear the nasal passageways and facilitate breathing, if your nose is congested. This method may not be a good idea if it's a foul smell that's triggering your gag reflex.

WARNING:
REMEMBER THAT THE GAG REFLEX IS YOUR BODY'S WAY OF PROTECTING YOU FROM CHOKING.

When disengaging the gag reflex with a toothbrush, don't start too far back. It is possible to desensitize a farther point in your tongue without first treating a spot toward the front and this isn't what you're trying to achieve.

CONSULT YOUR DOCTOR.
Excessive gagging could be a sign of a more serious condition, like GERD (Gastro Esophageal Reflux Disease), which has to do with your stomach and the acid levels in it.

CHAPTER SUMMARY

- The topic of Deep throating is so intense it had to get it's own chapter.
- The process of deep throating his penis is the complete turn on for him.
- When deep throating the penis you will inevitable encounter the dreaded gag reflex.
- The pharyngeal reflex or gag reflex (also known as a laryngeal spasm) is a reflex contraction of the back of the throat.
- Because our bodies are built for survival the brain will sense the trigger of your gag reflex as a call for help and in doing so will produce saliva in order to help free the throat from the obstruction.
- The top 10 ways you can reduce your gag reflex for a better fellatio experience:
    - **1. Numb your soft palate.**
    - **2. Disengage your gag reflex.**
    - **3. Relax**.
    - **4. Lift both of your legs if you're sitting or lying down on your back**.
    - **5. Make a fist.**

CHAPTER SUMMARY

- **6. Put a little table salt on your tongue.**
- **7. Hum.**
- **8. Listen to music.**
- **9. Beware the gag reflex in the morning.**
- **10. Breathe through your nose.**
- Warning: Remember that the gag reflex is your body's way of protecting you from choking.
- Consult your doctor. Excessive gagging could be a sign of a more serious condition, like GERD (Gastro esophageal Reflux Disease), which has to do with your stomach and the acid levels in it.

CHAPTER 9

"Flirting is a woman's trade, one must keep in practice."

— *Charlotte Brontë, Jane Eyre*

BEYOND SUCKING

Licking and nibbling is quite stimulating, so do it. Running your tongue around the glans, and then focus on the frenulum, this is his most sensitive part. Flick your tongue back and forth and all around the head of his penis while you are sucking, this will blow his mind. Don't forget to lick the bottom of his shaft while you slowing rub the head of his penis. Now with all this effort on your part is your partner quiet and even still? No worries. Pay no attention to his verbal cues but more to his no verbal gestures. Take a look at his testicles. When they are aroused they will rise up into his scrotum. So rather than hanging they will draw up like two scared cats pressed up against his thighs.

BE RESOURCEFUL

Try not to be miss bobble head. Do not simply move your head up and down on the shaft. Yeah you will get results but we are talking about giving a Rockstar blowjob, your skills must be advanced. Understand that your mouth and hands are more capable of providing different levels of pleasure than your vagina and anus.

Stick your tongue out and say "ah." Leave your tongue out of your mouth and use it to pleasure his tip as you stroke. As I mentioned before when you stick your tongue out to exhale you open your mouth wider. Although the shaft has less nerves that his tip, they sure do enjoy the sensation. Using your tongue and even lips will help to simulate him so intensely. Moaning when you do this will create a vibrating effect on his penis. Long before Hummer was a popular car, women were pleasing their partners by using this technique to send shooting stimuli though the bodies of men.

TRY SOME MOVES

Draw your lips into a tight circle, so there is almost a popping sound when the head moves in and out. WATCH YOUR TEETH! Once the action builds can easily cause injury if your not careful. However, some men like the feel if teeth and some even like for you to bite their penis. YES! "bite me bitch." Don't stop to look at him crazy that just what he likes and your there to please.

Try sucking his penis and creating a vacuum-like tightness and pressure. Don't be afraid to suck hard, as many men enjoy that strong sensation. Such on the head, or take the whole dick in your mouth and maintain the suction the entire time you slide it in and out of your month. Be open-minded and playful. As you practice you will find more way to please your partner.

GOOD VIBRATIONS

Add a little vibration to the your sucking. Yes you can hum on the penis but your mouth will never be as powerful as a battery. If you hold and bullet to your jaw while you suck you r entire head will vibrate. Vibrating cock rings are also a great way to provide this intense feeling.

Warning: Please don't keep a cockring on the penis for NO MORE than 20 minutes. The penis is exposed to extended periods of constriction can cause damage.

KNOCK AT HIS BACK DOOR

Many men enjoy anal stimulation. While your mouth is busy with his penis, gently touch his anus with the tip of your finger. If you get no kickback, insert that finger deep into his anus. If he response positively work that finger and your mouth and the same time. When your inside his anus you don't want to be to rough unless he wants you to. Search for his Prostate and add pressure. The Prostate feels just like the G-Spot on a woman and doesn't require much to stimulate it. Just press your finger upon it. He will respond to your advances, let him lead you. Use your other hand to press against the perineum, the area between the base of the penis and his anus. With these two areas stimulated you can bring great pleasure to his Prostate.

Many men are driven completely mad by this approach. If he enjoys rectal stimulation, you can take his dick into your mouth while facing him, then wrap your arms around his hips and use both hands to stimulate his rectum and anus. Hugging him towards you every time you take his penis deep into your mouth. Talk about multi-tasking.

THE CRESCENDO

By now probably you both have worked up a head of serious sexual steam and if your following the steps listed above you are a Rockstar Cockstar. If you feel he is approaching climax (i.e., his toes are curled, clutching the sheets, the neighbors know your name and he's proposed marriage a few time--a sure sign that you are doing things right), then you might want to slow down and let penis/vaginal action take place.

THE MOMENT OF TRUTH

Assume the position. Any position. When you sense he is ready to cum, quicken the pace. You should be pumping fast and furiously with your mouth and hands. DO NOT SLOW DOWN. You have to be totally committed at this point. Give him everything all at once. Head play, balls, anal, whatever it takes to get him to explode his load.

As he nears orgasm, you will notice changes. His breathing, quick and shallow; his muscles, tense and contracted; his balls, draw close to the body; his shaft, rock hard...KEEP PUMPING.

TO SWALLOW OR NOT TO SWALLOW

To Spit or to Swallow

- It's your decision: some like to take cum into their mouth, some like to watch it shoot. Both can be sexy.
- If you choose to take it in your mouth, you can swallow or keep a cloth or napkin nearby to spit into.
- Know your partner and make good choices. Swallowing during oral sex on a HOV-infected man can been know to transmit the virus

Most men enjoy it when you swallow their cum. Men who have strong feelings for their lovers in particular may report feelings of intimacy and acceptance when you swallow. Many find it difficult to swallow. Remember that its only a small amount of liquid, about a teaspoon or so. The taste of semen varies form person to person. If you don't like the taste change your partner diet. For which foods are best for a sweeter tasting cum go to www.learning.nikeemalee.com for my list of recommended foods.

If you find it difficult to swallow you may try holding your breath and swallowing quickly. Like taking a pill or medicine. Some people find it easier to deep throat at the point of ejaculation, this bypasses the taste buds.

If you find that none of these methods work for you, its ok. Just hold the cum in your mouth and spit it out or let him cum on your face or body. Either way he will be pleased with your experience and you will be a total Rockstar.

CHAPTER SUMMARY

- Licking and nibbling is quite stimulating, so do it. Running your tongue around the glans, and then focus on the frenulum, this is his most sensitive part.
- Try not to be miss bobble head. Do not simply move your head up and down on the shaft.
- Stick your tongue out and say "ah." Leave your tongue out of your mouth and use it to pleasure his tip as you stroke.
- Draw your lips into a tight circle, so there is almost a popping sound when the head moves in and out.
- WATCH YOUR TEETH!
- Try sucking his penis and creating a vacuum-like tightness and pressure. Don't be afraid to suck hard, as many men enjoy that strong sensation.
- Add a little vibration to the your sucking.
- **Warning: Please don't keep a cockring on the penis for NO MORE than 20 minutes. The penis is exposed to extended periods of constriction can cause damage.**

CHAPTER SUMMARY

- Many men enjoy anal stimulation. While your mouth is busy with his penis, gently touch his anus with the tip of your finger.
- The Prostate feels just like the G-Spot on a woman and doesn't require much to stimulate it.
- If you feel he is approaching climax (i.e., his toes are curled, clutching the sheets, the neighbors know your name and he's proposed marriage a few time--a sure sign that you are doing things right), then you might want to slow down and let penis/vaginal action take place.
- When you sense he is ready to cum, quicken the pace.
- As he nears orgasm, you will notice changes. His breathing, quick and shallow; his muscles, tense and contracted; his balls, draw close to the body; his shaft, rock hard...KEEP PUMPING.
- To Spit or to Swallow
  - It's your decision: some like to take cum into their mouth, some like to watch it shoot. Both can be sexy.

CHAPTER SUMMARY

- If you choose to take it in your mouth, you can swallow or keep a cloth or napkin nearby to spit into.
- Know your partner and make good choices. Swallowing during oral sex on a HOV-infected man can been know to transmit the virus
- Most men enjoy it when you swallow their cum.
- The taste of semen varies form person to person. If you don't like the taste change your partner diet. For which foods are best for a sweeter tasting cum go to www.learning.nikeemalee.com for my list of recommended foods.
- If you find it difficult to swallow you may try holding your breath and swallowing quickly. Like taking a pill or medicine. Some people find it easier to deep throat at the point of ejaculation, this bypasses the taste buds.
- If you find that none of these methods work for you, its ok. Just hold the cum in your mouth and spit it out or let him cum on your face or body. Either way he will be pleased with your experience and you will be a total Rockstar.

CHAPTER 10

"The best Pleasure is Self Pleasure

Nikeema T. Lee - American Author

SELF – PLEASURE

Self -pleasure is good for you and is considered to have actual health benefits. Self-pleasure is great; you get to do it by yourself, on your own terms, you can also experiment to find out what you like and what turns you on. Unfortunately growing up many people are raised with little information about our genitals and sex. Self-pleasuring does not really come naturally for everyone. The secret to bringing each person to orgasm is different. Women can climax through clitoral stimulation, vaginal penetration or G-Spot stimulation. There is no wrong way to self-pleasure we are all different. Here, in this article we will just try and point you in the right direction ladies.

SETTING THE MOOD

If you are going to get the most from the experience you must give yourself plenty of time. I would advise that you give yourself at least half an hour. Get yourself in a relaxed mood; take a bath or pour yourself a generous glass of wine. It is as much about state of mind as it is about technique ladies. Next make sure that you can't be disturbed. That means turning off the mobile/cell, locking the door and if you have children send them round a neighbors. Then get yourself in a position you feel comfortable and relaxed in. Women generally start out on their backs, legs bent and spread apart, with their feet on the ground. Make sure that you have plenty of support and cushioning.

FANTASIZE/ROMANTICIZE FOR SELF-PLEASURE

This is your alone time and recalling a past sexual encounter or elaborate on a favorite sexual fantasy can really set the mood. If you need a little of bit of help getting started then read an erotic story, look at a sexy publication or even indulge in a bit of adult entertainment. Ladies this is you time anything goes as long as it get the pulse racing.

EXPLORE ALL PARTS OF YOUR BODY

It amazing but a lot of women really don't know their own bodies at all. Experiment and run your hands all over your body and if some thing feels good then linger there and just enjoy the feeling it creates. Look at your genitals in a mirror (especially if you are unfamiliar with it) and caress the different parts to see what feels good to you. There are the inner and outer labia, your clitoris, your vagina and your perineum.

Don't be afraid to play around to find what is best for you

Ladies get those fingers working; use one or two fingers and start to stoke different parts of you vulva and remembering to stimulate your clitoris and labia. Find the rhythm that works for you this means experimenting with pressure, speed and motion. I suggest placing fingers either side of the clitoris and stoking up and down, or placing two fingers on the clitoral hood and rubbing in a circular motion.

LIFE IS ABOUT SURPRISES

Unless you are willing to open up your mind girls and let yourself be comfortable with your own skin and trying everything you will not get the most from your own body. When self-pleasuring try different types of touch: stroke, tickle, knead or why not even try gently pulling your genitals. Anything goes ladies. Use one or several fingers, the palm of the hand even your knuckles. Don't be afraid it will only take you to a better place.

IT IS A LONG AND WINDING ROAD

The thought of reaching that climax is all part of the fun. The thought of riding the wave will build the anticipation. You can add to that by enhancing the excitement yourselves girls. Learn to hold on to your sexual excitement by building up and then reducing temporarily the stimulus. Listen to what your body is telling you. Your own body will tell you when you have the right tempo or when a certain tickle feels good.

REMAIN RELAXED

As the sexual energy starts to build it is critical to let it take you and not to fight it. Breathing deeply rather than holding your breath will help as will rocking your pelvis as in intercourse will help. I would also suggest rhythmically clenching and releasing your PC muscle (if you are looking for vaginal penetration then a dildo will help).

RIDE THE WAVE

When the climax starts please continue to stimulate through the orgasm. The body starts to get more sensitive so lighten up during those first receptive seconds but keep going to enjoy the pleasurable aftershocks. The first orgasm may feel like a blip or an explosion however the more you practice the more range you will develop and understand.

Self-pleasuring is obviously a very personnel thing. It is something to be embraced and with practiced will only lead to a better orgasm as you find what works for you. Experimentation through self-pleasure will not only lead to personnel self-satisfaction but can only benefit your sex life as you work out what you like and then pass on that information to your partner.

CHAPTER SUMMARY

- Self -pleasure is good for you and is considered to have actual health benefits.
- There is no wrong way to self-pleasure we are all different.
- Set the mood- Get yourself in a relaxed mood; take a bath or pour yourself a generous glass of wine. It is as much about state of mind as it is about technique ladies.
- Fantasize/romanticize for self-pleasure -This is your alone time and recalling a past sexual encounter or elaborate on a favorite sexual fantasy can really set the mood.
- Explore all parts of your body
- It amazing but a lot of women really don't know their own bodies at all.
- Don't be afraid to play around to find what is best for you
- Life is about surprises Unless you are willing to open up your mind girls and let yourself be comfortable with your own skin and trying everything you will not get the most from your

CHAPTER SUMMARY

own body.
- It is a long and winding road The thought of reaching that climax is all part of the fun.
- Remain relaxed As the sexual energy starts to build it is critical to let it take you and not to fight it. Breathing deeply rather than holding your breath will help as will rocking your pelvis as in intercourse will help.
- Ride the wave - When the climax starts please continue to stimulate through the orgasm.
- Self-pleasuring is obviously a very personnel thing.

CHAPTER 11

"Good sex is like good bridge. If you don't have a good partner, you'd better have a good hand."

— Mae West, American Actress

THE BEST WAY TO MASTURBATE FOR MEN

This part is dedicated to the men who may have picked up this book. You too can be a Rockstar in the bedroom. Here you will learn the best techniques to self-pleasure and the key to elevating your sexlife to rockstar status. Now I know some of you reading this don't masturbate. Can you see me looking at you with the crazy eyes? I know. I have run across a few good men that just don't do it. Go figure.

So this section is anyone who was never taught the best way to masturbate. The thing is that oddly enough it's 99.99% of all men. Most men learn masturbation through trial and error, rubbing one out time and time again to find the best way to please him. You'll discover ways to give yourself more intense orgasms than you ever thought possible. And importantly you'll also find out how masturbation can make you a Rockstar at the real thing.

So ask the question. Do I need to masturbate in order to have a Rockstar Sexlife? Yes and No. No, because many guys end up having problems because they masturbate too much thus causing the ejaculation to become less intense and fewer. Yes, with the right techniques, you can develop the kind of sexual stamina that will leave women lying exhausted on the bed next to you. And even if you're not currently sexually active, the same techniques will give you stronger orgasms than you've ever had before.

MASTURBATION TECHNIQUES FOR MAXIMUM PLEASURE

THE BASICS – THE HAND

Most men learn early on that their hand is a friend with benefits. It's natural, effective and whole lot of fun. Yet many guys still get stuck thinking that the best way to masturbate is

simply as follows:
- Switch on a movie.
- Grip penis gently but firmly in your strong hand.
- Move up and down repeatedly at lightning speed.
- Ejaculate into a tissue or upon yourself, either way is fine.
- Return to the paused video game.

This is of course one of the most satisfying masturbation techniques known to mankind. The speed and pressure you can apply brings about a satisfying orgasm. But you can add much more variety as you'll see in the next few tips.

DON'T FORGET MADAM PALM'S TWIN SISTER: WAYS TO MASTURBATE USING YOUR OTHER HAND

Even at this basic level, you can still spice things up by using your other hand. Here are some ideas:
Try only using your other hand.
- Try using both hands at the same time. If you can put them one next to the other on your shaft, then lucky for you and any girl you meet. But if not, you can try placing the penis in between both

palms pressed together.
- You can use one hand to move up and down the shaft while the other plays with the head of your penis.
- Wringing is a great double-handed technique. Imagine wringing the water out of a cloth by squeezing your hands in opposite directions. Just be a bit more gentle with yourself!

DON'T LEAVE YOUR BALLS HANGING

Your balls are more than just an odd shaped storage facility. They are an erogenous zone which you can use to heighten your orgasms. It's up to you to work out the best way to masturbate by including your testicles; all guys are different, but here are some suggestions:

- Pull them slightly downwards while masturbating.
- Try caressing, stroking or tickling them – experiment to see what and where feels good.
- Try just holding them in a light but firm grip with the other hand.
- There is another good reason to spend some quality time with your balls. If you know what

they feel like normally, you can look out for any unusual lumps – something all guys should do on a regular basis.

IT'S NOT JUST WOMEN THAT HAVE MULTIPLE EROGENOUS ZONES

If you think the best way to masturbate is all about your penis, and maybe your balls, then think again. It's a popular belief that only women are blessed with multiple erogenous zones. But the truth is that men are more sensitive than you might think. For example try touching your nipples in the way that you would a woman's. Experiment with different strokes, pressure and movements. Try caressing the inside of your thighs or your stomach. If there's anywhere that you know you are sensitive, don't be afraid to explore yourself further with touch. Some guys will be more sensitive than others in different areas, so it's up to you to find out what works for you. There are no rules, so get to know your own body and find out what floats your boat.

MOVING SOUTH

The Perineum is the area in-between your anus and balls. It's a soft padded area which is sensitive to touch. You can try caressing it or pushing it gently with your spare hand.

The Male G-spot

Some cynical folk will say the male g-spot is a lost Atlantis which never existed in the first place. But there's no doubt that there are parts inside the anus which respond well to self-stimulation. For more open-minded and less squeamish guys, one of the best ways to masturbate is to include the anus. For others it's strictly a one-way street. If you're willing to explore here though, then you could be in for an orgasm-increasing treat. Here are some ideas for you:

Don't forget to wash before you start.

- Check that your chosen nail (yes – one finger will do) is short and not sharp. File it down if necessary.
- Add plenty of lubricant on your finger (proper lubricant is better so you don't accidentally stick something in there which can burn)
- Rub around the outside of your anus to begin with.
- Gently insert a finger as far as is comfortable.
- You can then just keep the finger inside while you masturbate with your other hand as normal, or move it gently in and out. Whatever works for you.

The G-Spot is a small area a couple of inches inside. It should feel like a little ball just over an inch in diameter. This is actually the outside of the prostate. You can softly rub this spot if you manage to find it, and if it's pleasurable.

Stimulating the G-Spot is known in the tantric sex world as a prostate massage, and is an effective way of enhancing orgasm. The key though with all these ideas is to be gentle and soft.

EXPERIMENT WITH DIFFERENT POSITIONS

If you just sit in your favorite chair or lie on your bed, you're not going to get anywhere near simulating sex. And as you'll find out in part 3, simulating sex is one of the most important masturbation techniques for men. Here are 3 ways you can use your body more effectively:

- Hold your penis under your body, lying on your bed on top of your hand. Then thrust into your hand.
- Try kneeling or standing and thrusting into your hand. The idea is to keep your hand still and use your body to move.
- Change positions from time to time: kneeling, standing, sitting, swopping hands or anything you can think of to add variety.

And in case you're wondering, unless you're a yoga master, have a missing rib or could enter the Guinness book of records for your length, it's extremely unlikely you'll be able to do the necessary gymnastics to use your own mouth.

SEX TOYS AND ACCESSORIES TO ENHANCE THE EXPERIENCE

The best way to masturbate without doubt is with a realistic vagina

I shouldn't need to point out the obvious difference between your hand and a real vagina. As I said earlier, masturbation isn't just about personal pleasure. It's also an investment in your ability to maximize both you and your partner's pleasure during sex. That's why simulating sex as closely as possible is an excellent way to prepare yourself for the real deal. It's also way more fun and intense than just using your hand. Anyway, we all know that many women use sex toys, so why can't guys too?

THE SLIPPERY JOYS OF LUBRICANT

For the same reasons that you would use a simulated vagina, lubricant is also an awesome addition to the repertoire of self-pleasure techniques. Whether you're using a toy or just your hands, lubricant will get you another important step closer to the real thing. A real vagina is wet and slippery, so a dry palm is a poor imitation of that amazing experience. Lubricant also makes it easier to stimulate the head of your penis, and of course explore your anus if you so desire.

THE DOUBLE-EDGED SWORD OF ONLINE MOVIES

Movies can be great if used the right way; they can also be damaging if used without any thought. As you'll find out in part 3, rushing masturbation can be a killer of your future sexual performance. And one thing which is sure to increase your arousal is your favorite movie. If you just switch it on, get yourself as excited as possible and rush to climax, you're unfortunately training yourself to be a future 'one minute man'. But if you use it as a tool when learning how to masturbate in a controlled way, then it's a great way to test your ability to keep relaxed and calm.

IMPROVE YOUR SEXUAL STAMINA AND ORGASM INTENSITY

Between 20 and 30% of men will suffer from premature ejaculation at some point in their lives. One of the main reasons guys end up having this problem is because of accidentally training themselves to climax very quickly when masturbating. But to give most woman an orgasm, on average you need to last for between 10 and 20 minutes during sex. So you also need to be able to last that long, and preferably longer, when masturbating. These next few sections will explain how you can achieve that. Please note though that if you already last for ages during sex, or when masturbating, there's no need to practice these.

But even though there is no need, some of these techniques can result in you having much more intense and powerful orgasms. This is for the simple reason that by forcing yourself to delay orgasm, it's usually more powerful when you do get there.

THE HUMAN TRAFFIC LIGHT: THE START AND STOP METHOD

In terms of techniques, the start and stop method is a really good way to masturbate. The simple version is that you set yourself a time, for example 30 minutes, and you don't allow yourself to ejaculate until that time is up.

Sound painful?

Well it can be, but not as much as the pain of the embarrassment of coming within 2 minutes every time you have sex.

KEGELS – RELAXATION AND THE LAST LINE OF DEFENSE

Kegels are a secret weapon you can develop in the safety of your bedroom. They can be used as a last line of defense to stop yourself ejaculating. But as well as strengthening the muscles for holding back ejaculation, they also teach you which body parts to keep relaxed during sex. In addition they're often used to get bigger and harder erections. And give you better bladder control when you've had too many beers. What's not to love about that?

BREATHE AND RELAX

This is more of a side dish to the main course of masturbation techniques. And again it's on the theme of learning self-control. Breathing slowly and deeply and keeping your body relaxed is a useful skill to learn when masturbating. The reason being that tension and over-excitement will extinguish your sexual performance faster than a fireman's hose on a wooden match.

CHAPTER SUMMARY

- This part is dedicated to the men who may have picked up this book. You too can be a Rockstar in the bedroom.
- Most men learn masturbation through trial and error, rubbing one out time and time again to find the best way to please him.
- The best way to masturbate is simply as follows:
  - Switch on a movie.
  - Grip penis gently but firmly in your strong hand.
  - Move up and down repeatedly at lightning speed.
  - Ejaculate into a tissue or upon yourself, either way is fine.
  - Return to the paused video game.
- Try only using your other hand.
  - Try using both hands at the same time. You can use one hand to move up and down the shaft while the other plays with the head of your penis.
  - Wringing is a great double-handed technique. Imagine wringing the water out of a cloth by

CHAPTER SUMMARY

squeezing your hands in opposite directions. Just be a bit more gentle with yourself!

- Don't leave your balls hanging
- It's not just women that have multiple erogenous zones
- Move south
- For more open-minded and less squeamish guys, one of the best ways to masturbate is to include the anus
- Experiment with different positions
- Sex toys and accessories to enhance the experience
- The best way to masturbate without doubt is with a realistic vagina
- Lubricant also makes it easier to stimulate the head of your penis, and of course explore your anus if you so desire.
- Movies can be great if used the right way; they can also be damaging if used without any thought.
- Improve your sexual stamina and orgasm intensity
- In terms of techniques, the start and stop method is a really good way to masturbate.
- Kegels – relaxation and the last line of defense
- Breathe and relax

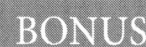

CHAPTER 12

"We waste time looking for the perfect lover, instead of creating the perfect love."

— Tom Robbins

HOW TO TANTRA

Tantra has much more to do with spirituality than sex. Although not generally considered a religion, it is an ancient non-denominational spiritual practice that evolved in India more than 7000 years ago. It was born out of rebellion against strict religions which denounced pleasure and reinforced the rigid caste systems that repressed virtually all personal evolution.

Tantra emerged so that the middle class could create a sense of spiritual and sexual freedom for themselves. Tantra has enjoyed more notice in the mainstream now than ever before (above and beyond Sting serving as its unofficial spokesperson), but it continues to be misunderstood by many.

Now, I cannot even begin to cover the details of the basis of general Tantra practice. However, I can give you a taste of the sexual component of Tantra so that you too can begin a path to enlightened sexuality and a Rockstar Sexlife. The sexual benefits of practicing some form of Tantra seems to be mind-boggling; from developing the ability to be multiply orgasmic (yes, men too); to the ecstatic energetic orgasms that last way longer than most of our measly 10 second experiences. Let alone the potential benefits of developing a true understanding of your own sexuality as well as an amazing bond with your partner.

BASIC INFORMATION
The main text of Tantric sexual practice is the Kama Sutra. The Kama Sutra reinforces the ideals of Tantric sex. Here are a few basic tenants of practice.

- Accept do not deny all of your sexuality.
- If it's consensual it is to be appreciated.
- Welcome, do not resist sexual energy.
- Enjoy what feels good without judging or

feeling guilty.
- Listen to your own heart and spirit.
- Sexual energy illuminates consciousness.
- Develop a sense of joyfulness in your life.

Tantra helps you shed your negative conditioning around sexuality. Many people suffer from those "guilt tapes" we play through our heads. Love and sex in this capacity are completely intertwined. That is why it is often referred to as sacred sexuality. Revere your lover and yourself as the amazing sexual being you are. Imagine yourselves as divine sexual deities. You do not have to be a couple to practice Tantra. There are plenty of ways you can develop your own sexual energy.

TECHNIQUES

Learn to meditate. Many of the techniques utilized require deep relaxation and an ability to be completely present minded - no focusing on work or the ballgame while having sex anymore boys and girls.

GET IN TOUCH WITH YOUR BODY.
Do yoga and learn to stretch. Many people walk around having no connection with their own bodies or what they are capable of. Movement is important whether it's belly dancing or learning to get comfortable in your own skin by learning to strip tease. You can even start by learning at home with The Art of Erotic Dance.

BREATHE.
It sounds simple but it's something we all take for granted at one time or another. Follow your own breath, deepen it; learn to coordinate it with a partner. Start by paying attention to how you breath when you're not in a sexual situation, then play with your breath during sex. Begin to breathe through arousal and orgasm. So many people have a tendency of holding their breath or breathing shallowly as they are about to come.

LISTEN.
The power of sound can be powerful; from healing to invigorating. And while sex is often peppered with groans and grunts, not enough people truly let their inhibitions go and vocalize during sex naturally.

TOUCH.

Re-program yourself to not just close the deal and move to the main event so quickly. This includes learning to touch other erogenous zones on your own body during masturbation. Fire in the Valley demonstrates techniques to use on yourself while Erotic Massage shows you how to connect with your partner through touch. You can also mix it up by varying your sensation. Try some Relationship Enrichment Massage Oil, or even better the Kama Sutra Love Essentials Kit provides you with a sampling of delectable treats to rub and lick off of your partner's body.

PC MUSCLES ARE YOUR FRIENDS.

It's been said again and again, the healthier your PC muscles are the better sex you'll have, the more bladder control, and potentially the easier labor will be for women. But men aren't left out of the loop either - it's just as important for them too. Kegel exercises are vital to Tantric sex. A Kegelcisor will come in handy as women begin to train these special muscles. Men can begin too by starting and stopping while they urinate. As well as experimenting with using their PC muscles to move their penises.

G-SPOT AND P-SPOT.

Get familiar with your G-Spot and if you're a guy it's time to finally say hello to your prostate. Both of these types of orgasms can really widen your sexual repertoire. Many people find these orgasms even more intense than clitoral/vaginal or penetration orgasms. Experiment on your own, so then you can introduce your partner to this type of play. And there are of course toys to help. Women can give the Waterproof Silicone G a spin and men and can try the popular Aneros.

Through these techniques you can learn to develop control over your orgasms. Many women tap into their ability become multiply orgasmic; while men can learn to delay ejaculation therein prolonging orgasms and becoming multiply orgasmic themselves (really, it's true!) You may want to also experiment with coordinating your orgasms with your partner (although it's not required).

CHAPTER SUMMARY

- Tantra has much more to do with spirituality than sex.
- The main text of Tantric sexual practice is the Kama Sutra.
- Basic tenants of practice.
    - Accept do not deny all of your sexuality.
    - If it's consensual it is to be appreciated.
    - Welcome, do not resist sexual energy.
    - Enjoy what feels good without judging or feeling guilty.
    - Listen to your own heart and spirit.
    - Sexual energy illuminates consciousness.
    - Develop a sense of joyfulness in your life.
- Tantra helps you shed your negative conditioning around sexuality.
- Learn to meditate
- Get in touch with your body.
- Breathe.
- Listen.
- Re-program yourself
- PC muscles are your friends.
- Get familiar with your G-Spot and if you're a guy it's time to finally say hello to your prostate.

CHAPTER 13

"No woman gets an orgasm from shining the kitchen floor."

— *Betty Friedan*

POSITIONS

Although positions are not the most significant practice in Tantra, the Kama Sutra does outline many positions that you can practice. However, keep in mind that they are most beneficial if you incorporate Tantric training. If you're in a coupled relationship, here are some options.

The Tripod While standing against or near a wall, the penetrating partner holds up one of the knees of the other partner firmly in one hand and then makes love face to face -- it then leaves the other hands free to explore and caress both of your bodies.

The Cat The partner being penetrated lies on their stomach while the other grabs hold of the ankles in their right hand, lift them high up and penetrates them, all the while rubbing their face, neck and chest with the other hand.

The Flower in Bloom The penetrated partner draws up both of their knees until they nestle the breasts; the feet rest in the other partner's armpits. The penetratee cups and lifts the buttocks with their palms, spreads the thighs and places the heels next to their hips, while the other partner caresses the breasts.

The Jewel Case The penetrator's legs lie along the other partner's legs, joining them from toes to thighs. One partner can remain below the other, or lie side by side. Another version of this position is to have your partner's thighs interlaced squeezing each other in a pulsating rhythm. This is called "The Squeeze".

Final Rule
Always be Grateful

ABOUT THE AUTHOR

Nikeema T. Lee, MS, wears a lot of interesting and important hats. Author, Intimate Relationship Coach, National Touring Artist and Certified Law of Attraction Guide. She is currently enrolled in a Ph.D. program getting her Doctorate in Holistic Counseling from the University of Sedona in Arizona.

Nikeema is on a national tour with the Pop Erotica Variety Stage Show "The Sweet Spot." As an Intimate Relationship Coach, Nikeema delivers a high energy erotic education segment to audiences across the country. She serves as a guide to helping people find the road to intimate self-discovery.

"My ultimate goal is to assist people on how they can become mentally, spiritually and emotionally free so they can have a great physical relationship."

"We are going to upscale our desires, take a lesson in understanding intimacy, while we eradicate self-destructive beliefs and behaviors," Nikeema says. "We can create the relationships we desire by having unconditional love and knowing true healing."

OTHER BOOKS BY THE AUTHOR

30 Days to Freedom: Becoming Authentic -2011

eBooks
The 7 Love Blocks -2014
Intimacy: Basic -2014

BROUGHT TO YOU BY
NIKEEMA LEE PUBLISHING HOUSE

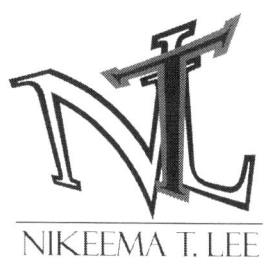

UPSCALE DESIRES

These exciting workshops are taught at the private location of your choice with special attention to your group's desires.

PRIVATE WORKSHOP THEME

HOW TO HAVE A BETTER INTIMATE RELATIONSHIP:

An interactive workshop that enhances communication and spiritual sexuality in relationships. Your will learn how to breath effectively during sex to achieve full spiritual orgasms as well as learning Tantric techniques.

HEAD OF THE CLASS:

Get top marks on pleasing your man. This workshop will prepare you for any pop quiz that may come up.

THE LINGUIST:

Become accomplished in languages of Cunnilingus and Pleasing your Woman. Every wanted to know just how your woman wants to be pleased...this one's for you.

ANAL 101:

no explanation necessary!!!

VIBRATORS 101:

Learn how to pick the right one to meet all your needs.

SQUIRTING AND G-SPOT

A workshop that is centered on developing techniques to female ejaculation.

SAFE SEX:

Learn how to play it safe and still have fun.

(This workshop is Free to youth organizations and non-profit groups that support at risk youths)

**TO BOOK YOUR VERY OWN
UPSCALE DESIRES EXPERIENCE
EMAIL: INFO@UPSCALEDESIRE.COM
WWW.UPSCALEDESIRES.COM**

HOW TO GET OVER A BROKEN HEART
HAS BROKEN HEART LEFT YOU LONELY?
MENTAL & EMOTIONALLY DAMAGED?
ARE YOU TIRED OF THE CHEATING?
TIRED OF GETTING HURT?

HEAL FROM HEART BREAK

Author & Intimate Relationships Coach Nikeema Lee has crafted a system that will give you;

- STRENGTH to move on or hold on
- COURAGE to love again
- WISDOM to learn from your mistakes

THE CLASS IS LIMITED.
WHEN YOU SIGN UP TO THIS DYNAMIC PROGRAM YOU WILL RECEIVE THE FOLLOWING;

Access to our 30 Day system, which includes.

- SUPPORT & Access to daily motivation affirmations
- REAL, RAW CONVERSATION
- GUIDANCE on how to Love unconditionally
- ENCOURAGEMENT

CHAPTER SUMMARY

Become Authentic and join this series on how you can CREATE a better you.

You are already great. Now reach, evolve and better yourself.

LIMITED SPACE AVAILABLE
Here's What is Included Your Package...

- Private 1:1 Coaching
- Heal from Heart Break Home Learning Program
- Guest Ticket for Heal from Heart Break Home Learning Program
- 3 Month subscription of SUPER EASY Moon Magic 28 Manifestation Program
- 3 Monthly LIVE Group Coaching Calls (
- Plus Free eBook 7 Love Blocks!

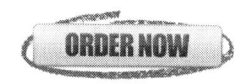

Coaching
www.NikeemaLee.com

Made in the USA
Charleston, SC
12 August 2015